Renal Diet Cookbook

The Comprehensive Guide For Healthy Kidneys – Delicious, Simple, and Healthy Recipes for Healthy Kidneys

Renal Diet Cookbook

© Copyright 2016 - All rights reserved.

The contents of this book may not be reproduced, duplicated or transmitted without direct written permission from the author.

Under no circumstances will any legal responsibility or blame be held against the publisher for any reparation, damages, or monetary loss due to the information herein, either directly or indirectly.

Legal Notice:
This book is copyright protected. This is only for personal use. You cannot amend, distribute, sell, use, quote or paraphrase any part or the content within this book without the consent of the author.

Disclaimer Notice:
Please note the information contained within this document is for educational and entertainment purposes only. Every attempt has been made to provide accurate, up to date and reliable complete information. No warranties of any kind are expressed or implied. Readers acknowledge that the author is not engaging in the rendering of legal, financial, medical or professional advice. The content of this book has been derived from various sources. Please consult a licensed professional before attempting any techniques outlined in this book.

By reading this document, the reader agrees that under no circumstances are is the author responsible for any losses, direct or indirect, which are incurred as a result of the use of information contained within this document, including, but not limited to, —errors, omissions, or inaccuracies.

Table of Contents

Introduction   VII

Chapter 1: What Is Renal Failure? How Does It Begin And Develop?   1
What Is Kidney Failure?   1
Causes   2

Chapter 2: Renal Failure Diet   5
What Is A Renal Failure Diet?   5
What Kind Of Changes Do I Need To Make On A Renal Failure Diet?   5
Foods That You Can Consume   7
Some Dietary Guidelines That You Should Follow   9
Risks Of Not Following A Renal Diet   9

Chapter 3: Benefits Of Having Healthy Kidneys   10
Regulation Of Water In The Body: 10
Removal Of Wastes And Maintains The Mineral Balance In Your Body: 10
Kidneys Also Produce Hormones: 11

Chapter 4: Lifestyle Changes   12
Lifestyle And Home Remedies   12
Prevention   13
Tips For Healthy Kidneys   14

Chapter 5: Breakfast Recipes   18
Quick & Easy Omelet   18
Healthy Whole Wheat Apple & Raisin Muffins   20
Delicious Apple & Cinnamon Crepes   22
Yummy Yogurt & Banana Smoothie   24
Tofu Berry Blast Smoothie   25
Bran Breakfast Bars   26
Fruity Yogurt "Lassi*"   28

Delicious Oatmeal & Banana Smoothie ... 29

Chapter 6: Lunch Recipes ... 30
Quick & Easy Mac 'N' Cheese ... 30
Chilled Rice And Apple Salad With A Honey Balsamic Vinaigrette ... 32
Creamy Baked Potato Soup ... 34
Barley, Beef & Potato Stew ... 36
Scrambled Egg & Green Onion Tortillas ... 38
Tangy Chicken Salad Sandwich ... 40
Delicious Bacon Topped Chicken & Corn Chowder ... 42
Asian Style Toasted Ramen & Sesame Salad ... 44
Creamy Tuna & Macaroni Salad ... 46
Sweet & Spicy Curry Salad ... 48
Refreshing Watermelon & Jalapeno Salad ... 50
Fruity & Chicken Salad With A Creamy Mayonnaise Dressing ... 51
Broiled Green Tomatoes & Goat Cheese Over Toast ... 53
Baked Herbed Chicken ... 55
Irish Style Baked Potato Soup ... 57

Chapter 7: Dinner Recipes ... 59
Stuffed & Baked Acorn Squash ... 59
Cottage Cheese Covered Baked Zucchini ... 61
Delicious Meat Stuffed Enchiladas ... 63
Baked Beets With Orange Zest ... 65
Berrylicious Wild Rice Salad With A Minty Dressing ... 67
Roasted Brussels Sprouts Tossed In Flavored Vinegar ... 69
Delicious Broccoli & Chicken Casserole ... 70
Chicken & Zucchini Lasagna With White Sauce ... 72
Delicious Low Sodium Surf And Turf Gumbo ... 75
Pan Cooked Chicken, Vegetable & Rice ... 77
Melt In The Mouth Crab Cakes ... 79
Sweet & Spicy Honey Mustard Chicken ... 81
Pickled Carrots With Dill Weed ... 83

Baked Fish With Lemon & Dill Weed 85
Zesty Grilled Chicken Kebabs With Lemon 86

Chapter 8: Dessert Recipes 88
Crunchy Popcorn, Pecan And Almond Caramel 88
Delicious & Nutty Baked Asian Pear Crisp 90
Fresh Blueberry Cheesecake 92
Quick & Easy Egg Caramel Custard 94
Chinese Style Vanilla Sponge Cake 96
Mint Infused Chocolate Cake 98
Quick & Easy Lemon Yogurt Parfait With Blueberries 100
Nutty Chocolate Fudge 101
No Bake Spiced Pumpkin Pie 103
Conclusion 104

Introduction

Kidneys are one of the vital organs present in the human body. It is important to ensure that they are healthy for maintaining your overall health and well being. This book will help you understand about the renal diet and different ways in which this diet will help you improve the health of your kidneys. The simple, delicious and healthy recipes in this book will help your kidneys stay healthy and strong.

To maintain healthy kidneys, the first step would be to understand what kidneys are, the benefits of having healthy kidneys, symptoms and causes of renal failure, the factors that put you at risk of renal failure, renal failure diet and the lifestyle changes that will help you in improving the health of your kidneys. Does all this overwhelm you? Well, you needn't worry. This book will guide you through all these steps! If you incorporate the suggested lifestyle changes then you will definitely see an improvement in your overall health!

To make it easy for you, we have collated a wide list of recipes that would benefit in controlling renal failure. These recipes are easy to cook and the ingredients are locally available. So, without further ado let's get started to understand what renal failure is and how you can detect and control it.

Chapter 1: What Is Renal Failure? How Does It Begin And Develop?

When the kidneys aren't able to purify and filter blood, it results in the accumulation of waste in the body, which is harmful for the body. This condition is referred to as renal failure and it can even cause death, unless treated on time. Before understanding what renal failure is, you need to understand what kidneys are. The two bean shaped organs that are located on either side of your spine in your back, are referred to as kidneys. They help in cleansing the blood by removing waste products from it in the form of urine. Not only this, but kidneys also help in maintaining the balance of certain elements in blood like sodium, potassium and calcium, and also control the secretion of hormones that help in controlling blood pressure and red blood cells.

What is Kidney Failure?

Kidney or renal failure refers to a condition where the kidneys aren't functioning like they are supposed to. "Kidney failure" covers a lot of different problems and some of these problems could be insufficient supply of blood to your kidneys for filtration. Diseases like diabetes, high blood pressure, any damage to the filters in the kidney can also severely damage your kidneys and any scar tissue or even kidney stones can block your kidney and result in renal failure.

There are different signs and symptoms that can help you spot kidney failure. It is important to be aware of these symptoms, because early detection can help in timely treatment and will curb the problem before it becomes severe. Keep an eye out for the following signs. If there is a decrease in the output of urine over a period of time, retention of any fluid that results in the swelling up of your legs, ankles or feet, extreme drowsiness, any shortness of breath, feeling of constant fatigue, confusion, seizures or even coma in some severe cases, build up of pressure in chest or chest pain. Also, there are cases where acute kidney failure that causes no signs or symptoms and can be detected through different lab tests that are done for some other reason. You should immediately take an appointment with your doctor when you start noticing any of the signs or symptoms of acute kidney failure.

Causes

There are different reasons that can cause acute kidney failure. These would include any condition that would slow down the supply of blood to your kidneys, any direct damage to the kidney or when the urine drainage tubes in the kidneys have been blocked because of the accumulation of waste in the body.

The first cause could be an impairment of the flow of blood to the kidneys and this could be caused due to different diseases and conditions like loss of blood or fluid from your body, use of medication for regulating blood pressure, heart attack and heart diseases, any infection, failure of liver, excessive usage of drugs like aspirin, ibuprofen, naproxen and other similar drugs, severe reaction to allergies, burns and excessive dehydration.

The second cause could be certain diseases, conditions and agents can cause severe damage to the kidneys and this would lead to acute failure of kidneys. Some of these diseases and conditions are mentioned here. If there are any blood clots in the blood vessels in and near the kidneys, blocking of the blood flow to the kidneys due to deposits of cholesterol, inflammation of the small filters present in kidneys, infection of any manner, destruction of red blood cells, lupus, particular medications like chemotherapy drugs, dyes that are used for testing and so on, cancer that targets the plasma cells, scleroderma, an blood disorders, inflammation of blood vessels in the body and the presence of toxins like alcohol, cocaine and even heavy metals can cause severely damage the kidneys.

The third cause would be the blockage of the passage of urine out of the body that can cause kidney failure. The conditions that can obstruct the passage of urine are bladder, cervical, prostate or even colon cancer, blood clots in the urinary tract, enlargement of prostate, kidney stones and any damage to the nerves that regulate the bladder.

Kidney failure usually occurs along with or due to another medical condition. There are certain conditions that increase the risk of kidney failure and these are as follows. If you are hospitalized for a serious condition that would require intensive care, age factor, blockages in blood vessels in your limbs, diabetes, kidney and/or liver diseases, heart diseases and high blood pressure are leading causes.

Chapter 2: Renal Failure Diet

What is a renal failure diet?

The main aim of a renal failure diet would be to control the consumption of protein and phosphorus in your daily diet. You would also have to start limiting the consumption of calcium, sodium as well as potassium. Renal failure diet can help you in decreasing the amount of waste that would be produced by your body, thereby decreasing the load on your kidneys and would definitely help them in functioning better. It will also help in postponing total kidney failure. Depending upon your health condition, your diet would also change. You might also need to make certain other changes to your diet as well if you are suffering from any other health problems like high blood pressure or even diabetes.

What kind of changes do I need to make on a renal failure diet?

The basic changes that you should make to your diet are as follows:

You will have to start limiting the amount of protein that you are consuming for decreasing the waste in your blood. You should reduce the consumption of foods that are rich in proteins like eggs, dairy products, meat, fish and poultry. You will also have to reduce the intake of phosphorus. When your kidneys are unable to get rid of the excess phosphorus, this leads to the buildup of huge amounts of phosphorus in your blood and this in turn would weaken your bones due to the loss of calcium. Food products like beans, dairy produce, peas, nuts and even whole grains are all considered to be rich in phosphorus. This is also found in beer, cola and cocoa. The intake of sodium needs to be cut down as well.

If you happen to have high blood pressure or if there are any extra fluids that are present in your body, then you will need to limit the intake of sodium. The intake of sodium on a daily basis needs to be cut down to 1500 mg per day. Avoid foods that are rich in sodium like processed and deli meats, sausages, canned foods, salted snacks, table salt and even soups as well. If your potassium blood levels are on the higher side, then you should also cut down on the intake of potassium. Limiting your intake of fruits and vegetables will help you in decreasing the level of potassium in your blood.

Finally, you will also have to start cutting down on the amount of liquids that you drink on a daily basis. If your body is unable to expel all the excess fluid, then this will lead to retention of fluid that will in turn cause swelling up and buildup of fluid in your lungs, thereby causing other health problems like shortage of breath.

Foods that you can consume

You should always ask your dietician about the amount of potassium, sodium, liquids and proteins that you should consume each day. Your dietician would suggest the serving size for the food groups that are mentioned below.

Starches: the following foods contain about 2 grams of protein, 80 mg of sodium, 35 mg potassium and 35 mg phosphorus. You can have a slice of bread, a small dinner roll or even a 6-inch tortilla, ½ cup of rice, cooked pasta, cereal, 1 ½ cup of unsalted popcorn, 4 unsalted crackers, unsalted pretzel sticks or vanilla wafers or 4 cookies.

Vegetables: One serving would contain about a gram of proteins, 25 calories, 15 mg of sodium and about 20 mg of phosphorus. Consume only fresh vegetables and not canned or frozen ones, because they have additional salt added to them. One serving would be equivalent to ½ cup. Green beans or sprouts, raw cabbage, aubergine, cucumber, onions, some corn, a cup of any type of lettuce, stalk of celery or raw carrot contain less than 150mg sodium. A serving of mushroom would have about 40 mg of phosphorus. One serving of broccoli or celery, mixed vegetables, snow peas, zucchini or summer squash would have about 150 to 250 mg of sodium.

Fruits: One serving of fruits would contain ½ mg of protein, 70 calories and 15 mg of phosphorus. Each serving would be equivalent to ½ cup. Apple juice, small apple, blueberries, cranberries, canned pears, grape juice or grapes, pineapple, strawberries, one tangerine or a serving of watermelon would contain less than 150 mg of potassium. Fresh peaches and pears, cherries, mango, small grapefruit or its juice or a mango would contain around 150-250 mg of potassium.

Dairy: The following products would have around 4 grams of proteins, 120 calories, 80 mg of sodium, 185 mg of potassium and also 110 mg of phosphorus. ½ a cup of milk, plain yogurt or fruit flavored, ice cream, buttermilk or chocolate milk, or one slice of cheese.

Nondairy substitutes: These foods tend to contain ½ gm of protein, 140 calories, 40 mg sodium, 30 mg phosphorus and 80mg potassium. A serving is equivalent to ½ a cup of nondairy frozen yogurt, creamer, dessert topping or a frozen dessert.

Meat and other protein foods: One ounce of cooked beef, pork or any poultry, one ounce of either frozen or fresh seafood like shrimps, lobster, fish, tuna, clams, unsalted sardines or salmon, 1½ ounce of crabs or oysters, 1 large egg or 2 egg whites would contain around 7 grams of protein, 65 calories, and approximately 25 mg sodium, 100 mg potassium and 65 mg phosphorus. Make sure that you don't add or use any salt while preparing these foods.

Fats: Fats tend to have very little protein and have around 45 calories, 55 mg of sodium, and 10 mg of potassium and 5 mg of phosphorus. You can make use of healthy fats like the unsaturated fats that are mentioned below. 1 teaspoon of margarine, mayonnaise, sunflower oil, soybean oil, olive oil, peanut oil, canola oil or 1 teaspoon of any oil based salad dressing like Italian or ranch.

Some dietary guidelines that you should follow

You might have to start taking different vitamin and mineral supplements because of the reduction in the amount of certain foods that you should consume. You should take vitamin supplements, if at all, according to the instructions given by your dietician. You should stop making use of any salt substitutes, because they contain potassium and this would again result in the rise of potassium in your blood. Always make sure that you are carefully reading all the nutrition labels on food before making a purchase.

Risks of not following a renal diet

The renal failure diet will definitely take you some time to get used to and it cannot happen overnight. If you simply cut down on the intake of food, then your body will be deprived of essential nutrients and calories that it requires for functioning. You will also start losing weight. If you do not follow a proper renal diet, then the stress on your kidneys will increase. This would cause total renal failure. If you have total renal failure then dialysis would become compulsory.

Chapter 3: Benefits of Having Healthy Kidneys

Kidneys are one of the most important organs in your body because of the three essential functions performed by them and these are as follows:

Regulation of water in the body:

If you want your body to function properly, then the water content in the body should be perfect. One of the main functions of kidneys in the body is the removal of excess water from the body or the retention of water when your body requires it.

Removal of wastes and maintains the mineral balance in your body:

All the substances that are present in the blood and also the other bodily fluids need to be kept at the required level if you want your body to function properly. For instance, sodium and potassium are two minerals that come from the food that you consume and your body needs these essential minerals for maintaining your health, but they need to be kept in the body at a certain level. Anything beyond or below this level would harm the body. When your kidneys are functioning properly, then the extra minerals, like sodium and potassium would leave your body in time, in the form of urine. The kidneys also help in regulating the levels of different minerals like calcium and phosphate that are very important for growth and developing the bone strength in the body. When your kidneys are function properly, they help in the expulsion of wastes such as urea and creatinine from the body. When your body breaks down protein that is consumed it results in the formation of urea and other waste by products. Creatinine is the waste product produced by muscles. When there's a renal failure, the levels of these waste products in the blood increase, because there is a decrease in the functioning of the kidneys.

Kidneys also produce hormones:

When kidneys are functioning normally, they also produce certain important chemicals, referred to as hormones. These hormones would circulate throughout the body and they help in regulating blood pressure, production of red blood cells and also the maintenance of the calcium levels in your body.

Chapter 4: Lifestyle Changes

Lifestyle and home remedies

When you are recovering from acute renal failure or when you are on a renal failure diet, then your doctor or dietician would recommend a particular diet that would help you in limiting the stress on your kidneys. Your dietician would analyze and then depending upon your current situation would suggest a diet that would reduce the pressure on your kidneys. Here are certain lifestyle changes that would help you in the recovery process and also help you to have healthy kidneys.

You should opt for foods that have a low level of potassium or no potassium at all. Foods that are rich in potassium are bananas, spinach, tomatoes, oranges and even potatoes. You can instead consume foods that have a low level of potassium in them like apples, cabbage, grapes, strawberries and green beans as well. You should avoid products that have added salt in them. You should cut down on the amount of sodium that you consume on a daily basis and this can be done by simply avoiding packed and canned foods, even frozen foods, you should also avoid processed meats as well as cheeses. Phosphorus is generally found in dairy products like milk, cheese and butter, also in beans and nuts. You will need to reduce the amount of phosphorus that you consume because this weakens your bones and also cause skin irritation. Once your kidneys start recovering, your diet would change but that doesn't mean that you should stop eating healthy foods.

Prevention

Renal failure is more often than not, difficult to predict or even prevent. But you can certainly lower your risk of renal failure by taking good care of your kidneys. Here are the things that you can keep in mind for taking good care of your kidneys. Whenever you are buying any over the counter medication, you should pay close attention to the labels. You should always follow the instructions that are given on these over-the-counter medicines like aspirin, ibuprofen and acetaminophen. Taking excess of the pain medication would increase the risk of renal failure and this is more likely when you already have any pre-existing kidney disease or any other problem like diabetes or high blood pressure. You should work along with your doctor for managing your kidney problems. Like mentioned earlier, if you have any preexisting condition or any other disease, then the risk of kidney failure increases. Especially when you have diabetes, high blood pressure or any other kidney related problem. Therefore you should stay on track with your treatment and follow the doctor's recommendations for managing your condition. You should make living healthy as your lifestyle choice and priority. Keep yourself active, stay fit by exercising regularly and eat a balanced diet and consume alcohol in moderation, if you drink.

Tips for healthy kidneys

You can do a lot of things if you want to keep your kidneys healthy and have them functioning properly. Here are certain tips that you can keep in mind for ensuring proper functioning of your kidneys.

Keep yourself hydrated:

You should always make sure that you are sufficiently hydrated, but you shouldn't overdo this. No studies have shown that over-hydration is good for enhancing the performance of your kidneys. It is definitely good to drink sufficient water and you can drink around four to six glasses of water per day. Consuming more water than this wouldn't definitely help your kidneys perform better. In fact, it would just increase the stress on your kidneys.

Consume healthy foods:

Your kidneys are capable of tolerating a wide variety of dietary habits and usually most of the kidney problems crop up from other existing medical conditions, like high blood pressure or diabetes. Because of this, it would be advisable if you were consuming foods that will help you in regulating your weight and blood pressure. If you were able to prevent diabetes and even high blood pressure, then your kidneys would be healthy as well.

Exercise regularly:

If you were already consuming foods that are healthy then it would also make sense if you were exercising regularly. Because regular physical activity will prevent weight gain and also regulate your blood pressure. But you should be careful about the amount of time you exercise or how much you exercise, especially if you aren't acclimatized to exercising. Don't overexert yourself if you are just getting started, because this would just increase the pressure on your kidneys and can also result in the breaking down of your muscles.

Be careful when making use of supplements:

If you are consuming any supplements or any other herbal remedies, then you should be mindful of the amount you are consuming. Consuming excessive amount of vitamin supplements as well as any herbal extracts can prove to be harmful to the functioning of your kidneys. You should talk to your doctor before you start taking any supplements.

Quit smoking:

Smoking causes damage to your blood vessels and this in turn would reduce the flow of blood to and in your kidneys. When the kidneys don't receive sufficient blood, they won't function like they are supposed to. Smoking also tends to increase your blood pressure and can also cause kidney cancer, apart from damaging your lungs.

Over-the-counter medication:

Whenever you are consuming any over-the-counter medications, then you shouldn't overdo it. Most of the common OTC medications tend to cause kidney damage if they are being consumed over a prolonged period of time. If your kidneys are healthy and if you consume these medicines for occasional minor ailments, then they don't pose a threat. But if you are taking them for any serious conditions like arthritis or chronic pain, then you should probably talk to your doctor before you start consuming them and you should also keep monitoring the functioning of your kidneys. If you know that you are a risk of renal failure, then you should keep getting regular screening of the functioning of your kidneys for making sure that they are functioning normally. If you have diabetes or high blood pressure, it is advisable that you get your kidneys screened for any dysfunction.

Keep a track of your nutritional values:

You should always keep track of what you are eating and also the serving size. You should keep a note of the nutritional values of the foods that you are consuming and discuss the same with your doctor.

Make use of meal-planning tools:

It might be tiring and troublesome to plan your meals for one day, let alone planning for an entire week. This would feel like a daunting task. You should make use of the online meal-planning tools or mobile apps that can help you plan your meals for the entire week without much difficulty. When you know what you are supposed to consume on a daily basis, then you can stock up on the necessary groceries for the whole week.

Read the labels carefully:

The next time you go shopping for groceries, make sure that you are reading the labels on food products carefully. Read the nutritional chart that's printed on the cover and if you don't recognize anything on it, then its better if you don't pick it up. You need to be very careful about the food products that you consume when on a renal failure diet.

Flavoring your meals without reaching out to the salt shaker:

You should monitor the consumption of sodium if you want to follow renal failure diet. A diet that is low in sodium will help in regulating your blood pressure and also will help you in fighting retention of fluids in your body. You can flavor your foods with spices, herbs and lemon juice instead!

Dining out:

If you know that you will be going out to eat then make sure that you have consumed as little sodium as possible during the rest of the day and opt for foods that contain less sodium when dining out.

Chapter 5: Breakfast Recipes

Quick & Easy Omelet

Serves: 2

Ingredients

- 1 cup filling of choice (chopped [& cooked if required] vegetables, cooked and shredded meats, chopped fruit or chopped [& cooked if required] seafood)
- 4 eggs
- 2 tbsp. margarine
- 4 tbsp. water

Preparation

1. Crack open the eggs in a large mixing bowl. Add the water, one tablespoon at a time, and whisk until well incorporated. Do not over whisk.
2. Place the margarine in a large non-stick pan and heat over a medium high flame until the margarine is melted and hot. The margarine should be hot enough to make a sizzling sound if even a drop of water is added to it.
3. Pour the beaten eggs into the pan.
4. Carefully, using a wooden spoon or a spatula, push the cooked edges towards the center of the egg so that there is space to push out the uncooked

portions onto the hot pan. Move the pan around so that the runny egg gets cooked.
5. Continue moving the pan around until the egg is well set and no longer runny.
6. Add the filling of your choice on one side of the omelet, taking care that the filling doesn't spill over onto the hot pan.
7. Carefully fold the omelet in half and serve immediately with some whole grain toast.
8. Enjoy!

Healthy Whole Wheat Apple & Raisin Muffins

Serves: 4

Ingredients

- 3 cups wheat bran
- 4 cups whole wheat flour
- 1 teaspoon nutmeg
- 2 1/2 teaspoons baking soda
- 1 teaspoon salt
- 2 cups apples, chopped
- 2 tablespoons grated orange rind
- 1 cup sunflower seeds or chopped nuts of choice
- 1 cup raisins
- 3 ¾ cups buttermilk or sour milk
- 2 oranges, juiced
- 1 cup molasses
- 2 eggs, beaten
- 4 tablespoons oil

Preparation

1. Turn on your oven and set the temperature to 350 F (about 175 C) and preheat for about 20 minutes.
2. In a mixing bowl, combine the wheat bran, whole-wheat flour, baking soda, salt and nutmeg together using a fork.
3. Add in the chopped apples, orange rind, sunflower seed or chopped nuts and raisins. Mix well.

4. Pour the juice from the two oranges in a measuring cup that is large enough to measure about 4 cups. Add buttermilk to it until the juice and buttermilk hit the 4-cup mark. (If you have a 2 cup measure, divide the juice in two and add in the buttermilk accordingly)
5. Pour this juice and buttermilk mixture to the beaten eggs.
6. Add in the molasses and oil and mix well to combine.
7. Pour the liquid ingredient mixture into the dry ingredient mix and stir well using a wire whisk to combine. Make sure there are no lumps.
8. Spray or grease a muffin tin with some oil and pour the batter into the muffin tin, until the tins are about two thirds full.
9. Pop the muffin tin into the preheated oven and bake for about 20 to 25 minutes, or until a skewer poked in the center of the muffin comes out clean.
10. Once done, allow to cool for about 15 minutes before removing from tin. Cool on a wire rack.
11. Enjoy!

Delicious Apple & Cinnamon Crepes

Serves: 2

Ingredients

- 8 egg yolks
- 1 cup sugar
- 4 whole eggs
- 2 cups flour
- 1 tablespoon salt
- 4 cups milk
- ½ cup oil
- 1 cup brown sugar
- 8 apples
- 1 teaspoon nutmeg
- 1 teaspoon cinnamon
- 2 stick butter

Preparation

1. To prepare the crepe batter, combine the egg yolks and eggs together in a bowl. Whisk until well beaten. Add the milk to the eggs and mix until combined. Slowly trickle the oil into the mix and whisk until combined completely.
2. Mix together the flour salt and sugar and combine using a fork.
3. Pour the wet ingredient mix into the dry ingredients and mix vigorously until it forms a smooth batter. Ensure that there are not lumps.

4. Heat a small non-stick pan over a medium high flame and spray with some oil.
5. Using a round spoon or a ladle, pour the prepare crepe mix on the hot oil covered pan and move the pan around to spread the batter in a thin uniform layer in the bottom of the pan.
6. Let the crepe cook for about 20 seconds before flipping it over using a spatula. Cook for another 10 second before taking it off the flame.
7. These crepes can be made up to a day in advance and should be stored in a cooler, covered with plastic wrap.
8. To prepare the filling, peel the apples, remove the cores and slice the apple into 12 slices each.
9. Heat a medium sized pan on a medium high flame. Add the butter to it.
10. Once the butter has melted, add in the brown sugar and lower the flame to a medium low. Allow to cook for a minute.
11. Add in the apple slices, nutmeg and cinnamon to the pan and toss well.
12. Continue cooking until the apple slices soften, but aren't mushy.
13. Take off the flame and cool to room temperature.
14. To assemble, place about 2 tablespoons of the prepared apple filling on one side of the crepe, but about an inch away from the edges.
15. Roll into a tight log.
16. Pop into the microwave or in an oven for a few minutes and serve warm with your favorite fruit sauce.
17. Enjoy!

Yummy Yogurt & Banana Smoothie

Serves: 2

Ingredients

- 1 large banana, peel removed and roughly chopped into large chunks
- 1 cup unsweetened applesauce
- 1 cup plain yogurt
- 1/2 cup skim milk
- 4 tablespoons oat bran
- 2 tablespoons honey

Preparation

1. Place the banana and the yogurt into the jar of a blender and blitz until smooth.
2. Empty the banana and yogurt mix into a large mixing bowl.
3. Add in the unsweetened applesauce and honey and mix well using a wire whisk.
4. Pour in the skimmed well and whisk well.
5. Pour the mix back into the jar of a blender and add the oat bran to it.
6. Blitz until thickened.
7. Serve chilled with some banana slice and an apple slice to garnish.
8. Enjoy!

Tofu Berry Blast Smoothie

Serves: 4

Ingredients

- 1/2 cup cranberry juice
- 1 cup raspberries, fresh or frozen
- 1 ½ cup silken tofu, firm
- 1 cup blueberries, fresh or frozen
- 1 teaspoon powdered lemonade
- 2 teaspoons vanilla extract

Preparation

1. Place the raspberries and blueberries in the jar of a blender and blitz until they get a smooth pulp like consistency.
2. Add in the silken tofu and blitz again smooth.
3. Pour in the cranberry juice, powdered lemonade and vanilla extract to jar and blitz again.
4. Serve chilled, garnished with fresh blueberries and raspberries.
5. Enjoy!

Bran Breakfast Bars

Serves: 6

Ingredients

- 1/2 cup oatmeal
- 2 ½ tablespoons diced medjool dates or coarsely chopped raisins
- 1/4 cup whole wheat flour
- 2 ½ tablespoons oil (safflower, soybean or corn)
- 1 1/2 tablespoons granular brown sugar
- 3/4 cup oat bran
- ¼ cup + ¼ cup boiling water

Preparation

1. Turn on your oven and set the temperature to 375 F (about 200 C) and let it preheat for about 20 to 30 minutes.
2. Place the diced medjool dates or coarsely chopped raisins in a mixing bowl and pour ¼ cup boiling water over the fruit. Let the water soaked fruit rest for about 30 minutes.
3. Mix together the oatmeal, wheat flour, granular brown sugar and oat bran together in a large mixing bowl using a fork.
4. Drain the fruit from the water and reserve the soaking liquid.

5. Add the soaking liquid to the remaining boiling water. Put this liquid in the blender with oil and blitz for a minute.
6. Immediately add the dry ingredients to the blender and blitz.
7. Pour the prepared batter from the jar to a mixing bowl and add in the soaked fruit. Mix well
8. Spray an oblong baking dish (10" x 8") with some cooking spray.
9. Pour the batter into the greased baking dish and level it with a spatula.
10. Using a knife, lightly mark the grooves for cutting: 3 columns and 4 rows. This will make about 12 bars.
11. Pop into the preheated oven and bake for about 25 to 30 minutes. Check the bars around the 20-minute mark to ensure that the bars are not burning.
12. After the bars are down allow to cool in the baking dish for about 10 minutes before unmolding and cooling on a wire rack.
13. Serve immediately or store in the refrigerator and serve chilled.
14. Enjoy!
15. (If these bars are to be kept for more than 2 days, it is advisable to freeze them, as these bars start getting mold quickly.)

Fruity Yogurt "Lassi*"

Serves: 4

Ingredients

- 2 cups plain yogurt
- 1 cup mango juice (or peach or apricot nectar)
- 1 cup milk
- 4 tablespoons, sugar (can be adjusted to taste)
- 1 teaspoon rose water (optional)
- 1/2 teaspoon cardamom (optional)
- 1/2 cup lime juice (optional)

Preparation

1. Beat the yogurt with a wire whisk until smooth.
2. Add in the milk and keep whisking until well combined.
3. Pour the yogurt and milk mix into the jar of a blender. Add the fruit juice or pulp of your choice, sugar and the rosewater, cardamom powder and lemon juice to the jar if you choose to.
4. Blitz until well combined.
5. Add some crushed ice to a tall glass and pour the "lassi" in it. Drink immediately!
6. Enjoy!

*A "Lassi" is typically an Indian sweet or savory beverage made using buttermilk or yogurt combined with milk or water.

Delicious Oatmeal & Banana Smoothie

Serves: 1

Ingredients

- 1/2 tablespoon wheat germ
- 1/4 cup oatmeal, cooked and chilled for a few hours
- 1/3 cup skim milk
- 1/4 banana, cut into large chunks and frozen
- 1 tablespoons brown sugar
- 1/4 tablespoon vanilla extract

Preparation

1. Place the cooked oatmeal in the jar of the blender and blend for at least 15 minutes or until it gets a smooth paste like consistency.
2. Add in the milk and blend again to loosen it.
3. Add the frozen banana chunks to the jar and blend again until smooth.
4. Finally, add in the brown sugar, vanilla extract and the wheat germ and blitz again until all the ingredients are well incorporated.
5. In a tall glass, add some crushed ice and pour the smoothie over it.
6. Serve immediately.
7. Enjoy!

Chapter 6: Lunch Recipes

Quick & Easy Mac 'N' Cheese

Serves: 4

Ingredients

- 1 ½ cups small pasta like, small shell, elbow macaroni or bowtie pasta
- 1 cup milk
- 1 tablespoon margarine or butter
- ½ teaspoon dry hot mustard
- ½ tablespoon chopped fresh tarragon or fresh thyme
- ½ teaspoon paprika
- 1 cup grated cheese, of your choice, can be a combination of two or more cheese too

Preparation

1. Turn on your oven and set the temperature to about 350 F (about 175 C). Let the oven preheat for about 20 to 30 minutes.
2. Heat a large vessel of salted water on a high flame. Once the water is boiling, lower to a medium low flame and add the pasta to it.
3. Cook the pasta until al-dente. Drain the water and dunk the pasta into a bowl of cold water. Drain and set aside.

4. Heat a small sauté pan over a medium high flame and add the butter to it. Once the butter has melted, add in the flour and cook until it forms a golden brown roux.
5. Once the roux is done, take the pan off the flame and slowly trickle in the milk and mix well. Be careful so that no lumps form, mixing well after each addition.
6. Once all the milk is added, return the pan to the stove and heat over a medium high flame until the sauce thickens. Keep stirring and scraping the sides to ensure that the sauce doesn't burn on the sides.
7. Add in the chopped tarragon or the chopped thyme, the hot mustard and paprika and mix well.
8. Add in the drained pasta and half the cheese and cook for a minute before taking it off the stove.
9. Grease a square 8" x 8" casserole baking dish with some butter or oil.
10. Pour the prepared pasta into the greased dish and top with the remaining cheese.
11. Pop the casserole into the preheated oven and bake for about 20 to 25 minutes or until the cheese melts and gets a golden brown hue.
12. Serve hot with some whole-wheat garlic bread.
13. Enjoy!

Chilled Rice And Apple Salad With A Honey Balsamic Vinaigrette

Serves: 2

Ingredients

- 1 cup rice, cooked and chilled (you can use any rice, but this recipe works best with white rice)
- 1/4 cup thinly sliced celery
- 1 medium apple or 2 small apples, chopped
- 1 tablespoon sunflower seeds, unsalted shelled
- ½ tablespoon olive oil
- 1 tablespoon balsamic vinegar
- 1 teaspoon honey
- 1 teaspoon orange zest, grated
- 1 teaspoon Dijon or brown mustard
- 1 clove garlic, finely chopped

Preparation

1. In a large mixing bowl combine together the chilled rice, sliced celery, chopped apples and the shelled sunflower seeds.
2. In a smaller bowl, combine together the olive oil, balsamic vinegar, honey, orange zest, mustard and garlic. Whisk well to combine.
3. Pour the prepared dressing over the prepared rice and apple salad and lightly toss to coat the salad with the dressing.

4. Serve immediately. If preparing in advance, cover the salad with a cling wrap. This recipe cannot be refrigerated or stored for more than 24 hours.
5. Enjoy!

Creamy Baked Potato Soup

Serves: 3 (makes about 1 ½ cup per serving)

Ingredients

- 1 large potato
- 1 tablespoon butter
- 1/6 cup flour
- 2 cups skim milk
- 1/4 teaspoon pepper
- ¼ cup shredded cheese (low fat)
- 1/4 cup fat free sour cream

Preparation

1. Turn up your oven to 400 F (about 200 C) and preheat for about 10 to 20 minutes.
2. Place the potato on a baking sheet and bake for about 10 minutes or until tender.
3. Remove from oven and cool.
4. Cut the potato lengthwise and scoop out the pulp using a spoon.
5. Heat a large saucepan over a medium high low and add the butter to it. Once the butter has melted, add in the flour and mix well.
6. Slowly add in the milk, stirring well to ensure there are no lumps. Keep stirring until it is well blended.
7. Add in the baked potato pulp and the pepper. Mix well.

8. Keep cooking until the soup thickens, stirring constantly to ensure that the sides do not stick and burn.
9. Add in the cheese and mix well until the cheese has melted.
10. Take the soup off the flame and add in the sour cream. Mix well.
11. Serve hot with a whole wheat bread toast.
12. Enjoy!

Barley, Beef & Potato Stew

Serves: 5

Ingredients

- 2 cups beef stew meat, cut into 1 inch cubes
- 1 tablespoon + 1 tablespoon olive oil
- 1/2 cup onion, finely chopped
- 1/4 cup mushrooms, thinly sliced
- 1/4 teaspoon garlic, minced
- 1/8 teaspoon dried thyme
- 1 cup low sodium chicken broth
- 1 1/2 cups water
- 1 cup mixed vegetables of your choice (such as carrots, French beans, peas, cauliflower, etc.)
- 1 potato, diced and soaked in water
- 1/4 cup barley

Preparation

1. Toss the beef cubes with the pepper.
2. In a large stew pot add 1-tablespoon olive oil and heat it over a medium high flame.
3. Add in the peppered beef cubes and sauté for about 5 to 7 minutes.
4. Add in the remaining olive oil.
5. Toss in the onion and mushroom and sauté again for about 5 to 7 minutes, stirring constantly.

6. Add in the thyme and garlic and sauté for a few more minutes, until the garlic and thyme are aromatic.
7. Pour in the water used for soaking the potatoes and the chicken broth. Mix well.
8. Finally add in the potato cubes, mixed vegetable and barley. Stir well and heat over a high flame until bubbling.
9. Reduce the heat to a low and cover the stew pot with a lid.
10. Allow the stew to simmer for at least 1 ½ to 2 hours so that the flavors can infuse well.
11. Serve hot.
12. Enjoy!

Scrambled Egg & Green Onion Tortillas

Serves: 2

Ingredients

- 2 corn tortillas, about 6 inches in diameter
- 1/4 tablespoon olive oil
- 2 scallions (green onions), thinly sliced
- 1/4 of pepper red bell pepper, finely diced
- 2 eggs, beaten

Preparation

1. Pour the oil into a medium sized frying pan and heat over a medium low flame.
2. Add in the green onions and red bell pepper and sauté for about 5 minutes, or until the vegetables are tender, but firm.
3. Pour in the eggs and scramble using a wire whisk. Cook for about 5 more minutes or until the eggs are completely cooked.
4. Take two clean kitchen towels and dampen them. Wring out the excess water. Place the tortilla between the two towels and then place it on a plate.
5. Microwave on medium heat for about 2 to 3 minutes. Repeat with second tortilla.
6. Divide the prepared egg mixture between the two tortillas and roll them up tightly into logs.
7. Serve immediately.

8. Enjoy!

Tangy Chicken Salad Sandwich

Ingredients

Serves: 3

- ½ tablespoon olive oil
- ½ teaspoon pepper
- 1/2 cup boneless and skinless chicken breast, chopped into bite sized portions
- 1/4 cup green pepper, cut into ½ inch cubes
- 1/4 cup celery, diced
- 1/8 cup onion, finely sliced
- 1/2 cup mandarin oranges (peel and chop them into bite sized portions)
- 1/6 cup mayonnaise
- 6 slices of bread of your choice (or you can ditch the bread and just have the salad!)

Preparation

1. Pour the oil into a medium sized sauté pan and heat it over a medium low flame. Add in the chicken and the pepper and toss well until cooked. Drain and set aside.
2. Place the green pepper, cooked chicken, celery and onion together in a bowl and mix well using a wooden spoon.
3. Add in the mandarin orange bites and the mayonnaise and mix well to combine. Do not mix too vigorously.

4. Spoon the salad onto a slice of bread and cover with another slice.
5. Serve immediately.
6. Enjoy!

Delicious Bacon Topped Chicken & Corn Chowder

Serves: 6

Ingredients

- 5 slices of bacon, low sodium
- 1 onion, finely chopped
- 4 green onions (scallions), finely chopped
- 3 ½ cups low sodium chicken broth
- 4 cups corn
- 2 potatoes, diced and soaked in water
- 4 boneless and skinless chicken breasts, diced
- 2 cups whipping cream
- 3 tablespoons fresh thyme, finely chopped
- 1 teaspoon crushed black pepper

Preparation

1. Place the bacon strips in a large pan and cook until crisp. Drain the bacon from the fat and set aside.
2. Add the onion to the bacon fat and sauté until the onions are translucent.
3. Pour in the broth and the potatoes (along with the soaking liquid).
4. Cover the pan and reduce the heat. Allow the broth to simmer for at least 15 minutes.
5. Add in the corn, chicken and thyme.
6. Cover again and let the broth simmer for another 15 minutes so that the chicken is cooked through.

7. Add in the whipping cream and heat for another 2 minutes.
8. Take off heat and pour into individual soup bowls.
9. Serve hot topped with the prepared bacon (crumbled), a sprinkle of crushed black pepper and a healthy helping of crispy scallions.
10. Enjoy!

Asian Style Toasted Ramen & Sesame Salad

Serves: 4

Ingredients

- 1 cup boneless and skinless chicken or turkey, cooked and diced
- 1/4 head cabbage, finely shredded
- 2 green onions, diced
- 1 package ramen noodles
- 1 tablespoon sesame seeds
- 1/2 tablespoon olive oil
- 1/4 cup rice vinegar or white wine vinegar
- 1/2 tablespoon sesame oil
- 1/8 cup sugar
- 1 tablespoon olive oil

Preparation

1. Smash the ramen noodles into small bits while still in the package. Open the packet and take the seasoning packet out.
2. Pour ½ tablespoon olive oil into a pan and heat over a medium low flame.
3. Add in the crushed noodles and the sesame seeds.
4. Cook until they get a golden brown hue, stirring constantly to ensure that neither the noodles nor the sesame seeds burn.

5. Combine together the cooked chicken (or the turkey), finely shredded cabbage and the onions in a large mixing bowl. Add the contents of the pan to the mixing bowl and mix well.
6. In a small mixing bowl combine together the remaining olive oil, rice vinegar (or white wine vinegar), sesame oil and sugar together. Whisk well to combine.
7. Pour the dressing onto the salad and toss well to coat.
8. Serve immediately.
9. Enjoy!

Creamy Tuna & Macaroni Salad

Serves: 2 (1 cup per serving)

Ingredients

- 6 tablespoons cup mayonnaise
- 3/4 cups shell macaroni
- 1 tablespoon vinegar
- 1/2 can unsalted tuna, 6 ½ ounce can, drained, chopped into bite sized pieces (can also use water packed tuna)
- 1/4 cup celery, finely chopped
- 1/4 cup peas, lightly boiled
- 1/2 tablespoon dried dill

Preparation

1. Heat a large vessel of salted water on a high flame. Once the water is boiling, lower to a medium low flame and add the pasta to it.
2. Cook the pasta until al-dente. Drain the water and dunk the pasta into a bowl of cold water. Drain and set aside.
3. Combine the mayonnaise and vinegar in a large mixing bowl and whisk well to combine.
4. Add in the tuna pieces, celery, peas and dill. Mix well.
5. Add the shell macaroni and mix lightly to ensure that the pasta doesn't break.
6. Cover the bowl with a cling film and refrigerate.

7. Serve chilled.
8. Enjoy!

Sweet & Spicy Curry Salad

Serves: 4

Ingredients

- 1 cup chicken or turkey, cut into bite sized pieces
- 6 tablespoons light sour
- 6 tablespoons mayonnaise
- 1/4 cup mango chutney
- 1/4 cup nuts, finely sliced (you can use almonds, pecans or cashew nuts)
- 2 stalks celery, chopped
- 1 tablespoon curry powder
- 2 green onions (scallions), chopped
- 1/4 cup raisins
- ½ teaspoon crushed black pepper
- ½ tablespoon olive oil

Preparation

1. Heat the olive oil in a sauté pan over a medium high flame. Add the chopped chicken or turkey to the pan and sprinkle crushed black pepper over it.
2. Cook for about 5 minutes, stirring constantly, until the meat is cooked. Drain and set aside.
3. In a small mixing bowl combine the curry powder, mayonnaise, light sour and mango chutney together to form a dressing. Set aside.

4. In a large mixing bowl, combine together the cooked chicken (or turkey), sliced nuts, celery, green onions, and raisins. Mix well.
5. Pour the dressing over the prepared salad and toss well to coat.
6. Cover the salad with a cling film and refrigerate overnight.
7. Serve chilled.
8. Enjoy!

Refreshing Watermelon & Jalapeno Salad

Serves: 3

Ingredients

- 1 1/2 cup watermelon, chopped into bite sized chunks, seeds removed
- 1 tablespoon lime juice
- 1/2 cup green bell pepper, finely chopped
- 1/2 tablespoon cilantro, finely chopped
- 1 medium jalapeno, cut length wise, seeds removed and minced
- 1/2 tablespoon green onion, chopped
- 1 garlic clove, crushed

Preparation

1. In a large mixing bowl combine together the watermelon chunks, green bell pepper, jalapeno, green onion and garlic. Mix well.
2. Pour the lemon juice over the prepared salad and toss well to coat.
3. Cover the bowl with a cling film and refrigerate for at least 2 hours.
4. Serve chilled topped with cilantro.
5. Enjoy!

Fruity & Chicken Salad With A Creamy Mayonnaise Dressing

Serves: 2

Ingredients

- 1 cup chicken breasts, chopped into bite sized pieces
- ½ tablespoon olive oil
- ½ teaspoon pepper
- 2 cups radiatore pasta
- 1/2 stalk celery, finely chopped
- 1/2 cup brown almonds, silvered
- 1/2 green onion (scallions), finely chopped
- 1/2 apple, cubed
- 1 cup seedless grapes, cut into quarters
- 6 tablespoons raisins
- 1 tablespoon 5 spice powder
- ½ cup mayonnaise
- 4 tablespoons rice vinegar
- ½ cup sour cream
- 2 tablespoons sugar

Preparation

1. Heat the olive oil in a sauté pan over a medium high flame. Add the chopped chicken or turkey to the pan and sprinkle crushed black pepper over it.
2. Cook for about 5 minutes, stirring constantly, until the meat is cooked. Drain and set aside.

3. Heat a large vessel of salted water on a high flame. Once the water is boiling, lower to a medium low flame and add the pasta to it.
4. Cook the pasta until al-dente. Drain the water and dunk the pasta into a bowl of cold water. Drain and set aside.
5. Combine the cooked chicken, cooked pasta, celery, silvered almonds, green onion, apple, grapes and raisins together in a large mixing bowl.
6. To prepare the dressing, combine together the sour cream, mayonnaise, sugar, rice vinegar and 5-spice powder in a medium mixing bowl. Whisk well to combine.
7. Cover the bowl with a cling film and refrigerate for at least 2 hours.
8. Serve chilled.
9. Enjoy!

Broiled Green Tomatoes & Goat Cheese Over Toast

Serves: 2

Ingredients

- 2 medium green tomatoes
- 1 teaspoon oregano leaves, finely chopped
- 1/2 tablespoon balsamic vinegar
- 1/2 cup goat cheese, crumbled
- Ground black pepper, to taste
- 2 teaspoons olive oil
- 4 slices French bread, toasted

Preparation

1. Chop the green tomatoes into ½ inch thick slices.
2. Pour a little olive oil into a shallow baking dish and swivel it around so that the baking dish is well coated with oil.
3. Place the tomato slices in a single overlapping layer in the bottom of the greased baking dish.
4. Drizzle the vinegar over the tomato slices and sprinkle the finely chopped oregano over them.
5. Add the crumbled goat cheese and drizzle the remaining olive oil over the goat cheese.
6. Place the baking dish in a preheated oven and broil about 5 to 8 inches below the broiler, for about 8 to10 minutes or until the tomatoes get hot and the

cheese has melted and starts to brown around the edges.
7. Remove the baking dish from the oven and allow it to cool for a few minutes. Carefully spoon out the prepared tomato and cheese and place it on the toasted bread. Sprinkle some pepper over it.
8. Serve immediately.
9. Enjoy!

Baked Herbed Chicken

Serves: 2

Ingredients

- 1/2 pound skinless & boneless chicken breasts, or 3/4 pound chicken with bone
- 1 slice whole wheat bread
- 1/4 teaspoon fresh thyme
- 1/4 teaspoon fresh basil
- 1/4 teaspoon fresh ground black pepper
- 1/4 teaspoon fresh tarragon
- 1/4 teaspoon fresh paprika
- 1/4 teaspoon fresh oregano

Preparation

1. Turn up your oven to 400 F (about 200 C) and preheat for about 10 to 20 minutes.
2. In the jar of a blender or a food processor, place the whole wheat bread, thyme, basil, ground black pepper, tarragon, paprika and oregano.
3. Blitz until well combined.
4. Dunk the chicken in a bowl of chilled water and immediately dip it in the bread, herb and spice mix.
5. Grease a shallow baking dish with some oil and place the herb crusted chicken in the baking dish.
6. Pop the baking dish into the preheated oven and bake for about 25 to 30 minutes (if using boneless

chicken) or about 55 minutes to an hour (if using chicken with bone).
7. Remove from the oven and allow the chicken to rest for a few minutes.
8. Serve hot with a side of boiled vegetables and a sauce of your choice.
9. Enjoy!

Irish Style Baked Potato Soup

Serves: 3

Ingredients

- 2 ounces cheese, cubed or grated
- 1 large potato, if available, use a Russet potato
- 2 cups skim milk
- 2 ½ cups flour
- 1/2 teaspoon ground black pepper
- 1/4 cup fat free sour cream

Preparation

1. Turn up your oven to 400 F (about 200 C) and preheat for about 10 to 20 minutes.
2. Place the potato on a baking sheet and pop into the preheated oven for about 10 minutes or until the center is soft, yet firm.
3. Once down, remove from the oven and allow the potato to cool. Once cool, slice the potato lengthwise and scoop out the pulp using a spoon.
4. In a large saucepan, add the flour and slowly add the milk to the flour, stirring constantly until the flour and milk are well combined.
5. Add in the ground black pepper and the potato pulp.
6. Heat the pan over a medium high flame and cook until the soup thickens and starts bubbling.
7. Add in the cheese and stir constantly until the cheese melts.

8. Remove the soup from heat and pour into individual bowls.
9. Serve immediately topped with about a teaspoon of grated cheese.
10. Enjoy!

Chapter 7: Dinner Recipes

Stuffed & Baked Acorn Squash

Serves: 1

Ingredients

- 1/2 acorn squash, cut length wise, seeds removed
- 1/2 tablespoon butter or margarine
- 1 teaspoon brown sugar
- 1 teaspoon butter or margarine
- 1 1/2 tablespoon pineapple, crushed
- 1 teaspoon nutmeg, powdered

Preparation

1. Turn up your oven to 400 F (about 200 C) and preheat for about 10 to 20 minutes.
2. Grease a baking pan and place the slice of squash with its cut side up.
3. Rub one-teaspoon butter or margarine on the acorn half and sprinkle the brown sugar over it.
4. Pop the baking dish into the preheated oven and bake for at least 30 to 35 minutes or until the squash is tender.
5. Once the squash is done, remove from the oven and cool to room temperature.
6. Crank up the oven to 425 F (about 220 C) and leave it on.

7. Spoon out the pulp from the squash, making sure that you leave behind a sturdy shell behind that is at least ¼ inch thick.
8. In a small mixing bowl, combine together the cooked acorn squash pulp, the remaining butter, nutmeg powder and the crushed pineapple and mix well.
9. Spoon this mixture into the shell and place the filled acorn squash shells onto the greased baking dish.
10. Pop the baking dish bake into the preheated oven and bake for another 15 minutes.
11. Serve hot.
12. Enjoy!

Cottage Cheese Covered Baked Zucchini

Serves: 3

Ingredients

- 3 medium sized zucchini, sliced lengthwise
- 1/8 cup parsley, finely chopped
- 1/8 cup grated parmesan cheese
- 1/4 cup finely chopped onion
- 2 sticks celery, finely chopped
- 3/4 cup low fat cottage cheese
- 1 tablespoon margarine or butter
- 3 tablespoons buttermilk
- 1/8 teaspoon ground black pepper
- 1 egg, beaten well
- 1/2 teaspoon oregano
- 3 teaspoons grated cheese (1/2 teaspoon for each zucchini halve), for garnish

Preparation

1. Turn up your oven to 350 F (about 175 C) and preheat for about 10 to 20 minutes.
2. In a small sauté pan add the butter or margarine and heat over a medium low flame.
3. Add in the onion and celery and sauté for about 5 minutes or until tender.
4. Crumble or grate the cottage cheese and add into the pan. Cook for about 2 minutes.

5. Combine the buttermilk, ground black pepper, egg and oregano and add to the pan. Mix well.
6. Add in the parsley and cook for a minute more and take off heat.
7. Place the zucchini slices in a greased baking dish with the cut side up and cover the baking dish with aluminum foil.
8. Pop the covered baking dish into the preheated oven and bake for about 15 minutes.
9. Spread the prepared cottage cheese mixture on the zucchini halves and bake again uncovered for another 15 minutes or until done.
10. Sprinkle with cheese and serve immediately.
11. Enjoy!

Delicious Meat Stuffed Enchiladas

Serves: 3

Ingredients

- 1/2 pound lean ground beef or minced chicken breast
- 1/2 can enchilada sauce
- 2 cloves garlic, finely chopped
- 1/4 cup onion, finely chopped
- 6 corn tortillas
- ½ teaspoon cumin
- ½ teaspoon ground black pepper
- Olive oil, for frying
- 1 cup mixed carrots, cucumber and beetroot sticks, soaked in vinegar

Preparation

1. Turn up your oven to 375 F (about 190 C) and preheat for about 10 to 20 minutes.
2. Heat a medium sized frying pan on a medium high flame. Add in the ground beef or minced chicken and cook until well browned.
3. Add in the chopped garlic, chopped onion, and cumin and ground black pepper.
4. Continue cooking until the onion is tender.
5. In another pan, add very little olive oil and lightly fry the tortillas.

6. Spread about a tablespoon of the enchilada sauce on each tortilla.
7. Spoon the mixture onto the prepared tortilla and top with the vinegar soaked vegetables.
8. Roll into a tight log.
9. You can lightly fry the enchiladas again for a crispy exterior.
10. Serve immediately with a side of sliced olives, vinegar soaked veggies and a sauce of your choice.
11. Enjoy!

Baked Beets With Orange Zest

Serves: 2

Ingredients

- 1/2 bunch red beets
- 1/2 teaspoon olive oil
- 1/2 teaspoon red wine vinegar
- 1/4 teaspoon orange zest, grated

Preparation

1. Turn up your oven to 400 F (about 200 C) and preheat for about 10 to 20 minutes.
2. Thoroughly wash the beets, getting rid of all the dirt and grime. Remove the tops off the beets, but leave on about ½ inch of the stem.
3. Loosely wrap the beets up in a large foil and place them on a baking sheet.
4. Pop the baking sheet into the preheated oven and bake for about 50 minutes to an hour or until the beets are tender.
5. Remove from the oven and cool before removing the foil off the beets.
6. Peel the cooled down beets and trim the tops and their tails.
7. Chop the beets into halves or quarters, as per their size.
8. Add the vinegar and toss well. Refrigerate for a few hours so that the beets marinate well.

9. Just before serving, drizzle the olive oil over the marinated beets and add in the orange zest.
10. Toss well and serve immediately.
11. Enjoy!

Berrylicious Wild Rice Salad With A Minty Dressing

Serves: 4

Ingredients

- 1/2 cup uncooked wild rice
- 1/2 cup collard greens, lightly steamed
- 1 cup water
- 1/4 cup onion, chopped
- 1/8 cup blueberries
- 1 1/4 cups mixed berries, like blueberries, blackberries, raspberries, etc.)
- 1 tablespoon lemon juice
- 1/2 tablespoon olive oil
- 1/8 cup fresh mint, finely chopped
- 1/4 cup fat free or low fat sour cream

Preparation

1. Rinse the rice well and place in a large saucepan. Pour the water over the rice.
2. Heat over a high flame until the water starts bubbling. Once boiling, lower the heat and cover the saucepan. Let the water simmer for about 50 minute to an hour or until most of the liquid is absorbed.
3. Empty the cooked rice into a large mixing bowl and add in the steamed collard greens, onion and the mixed berries. Mix well.

4. In the jar of a blender or a food processor, add in the lemon juice, olive oil and mint leaves. Blitz until it gets a smooth paste like consistency. Add in a little water if the paste is too thick or gunky.
5. Pour the dressing into a medium sized mixing bowl and slowly add in the sour cream, whisking vigorously while you pour.
6. Pour the prepared dressing over the salad and toss well to coat.
7. Serve immediately topped with the 1/8-cup blueberries.
8. If you wish to store the salad, cover the bowl with a cling film and refrigerate to keep it fresh and add the blueberries later.
9. Enjoy!

Roasted Brussels Sprouts Tossed In Flavored Vinegar

Serves: 2

Ingredients

- 1 cup Brussels sprouts
- 2 tablespoons olive oil
- 2 tablespoons herb or fruit flavored vinegar
- 2 tablespoons fresh parmesan cheese, grated

Preparation

1. Turn up your oven to 450 F (about 220 C) and preheat for about 10 to 20 minutes.
2. Chop the larger sprouts into halves, while leaving the smaller sprouts whole.
3. Sprinkle the olive oil over the Brussels sprouts and toss with your hands to coat well.
4. Place the Brussels sprouts coated in oil on a lightly oiled baking sheet.
5. Pop it in the preheated oven and bake for about 15 minutes, or till the sprouts are tender. Check the sprouts by piercing them with a fork.
6. Remove the sprouts from the oven and drizzle the herb or fruit vinegar on the roasted sprouts. Toss well.
7. Top with the grated Parmesan cheese and serve immediately.
8. Enjoy!

Delicious Broccoli & Chicken Casserole

Serves: 3

Ingredients

- 1 cup grated cheese
- 1 1/2 cups broccoli florets
- 1 1/2 chicken breast, diced
- 1 small onion, chopped
- 1 tablespoon margarine or butter
- 1 cup milk
- 1 egg, beaten
- 1 cup barley, rice or noodles, cooked
- Grated parmesan, to top

Preparation

1. Turn up your oven to 350 F (about 175 C) and preheat for about 10 to 20 minutes.
2. Fill a vessel with water and heat on a high flame until bubbling. Add the broccoli florets to the bubbling water and cook on high flame for about 5 minutes or until tender. Drain from the water and dunk into cold water. Drain and set aside.
3. In a sauté pan add the butter or margarine and heat on a medium low flame. Once melted, add in the chicken pieces and onion and cook until the chicken is well browned and the onion is tender. Drain and set aside.

4. In a large mixing bowl, combine together the cooked broccoli florets, cooked chicken, milk, beaten egg, grated cheese and cooked barley, rice or noodles. Mix lightly.
5. Pour the prepared mix into a greased casserole baking dish.
6. Sprinkle the grated Parmesan cheese in a thin layer.
7. Pop into the preheated oven and back for about 1 hour and 20 to 30 minutes or until it is set and a skewer or fork inserted in the center comes out clean.
8. Remove from the oven and let it cool for a few minutes.
9. Serve hot with a side of toasted whole wheat bread.
10. Enjoy!
11. Cook broccoli in microwave.
12. Meanwhile, brown onion and chicken in butter in a pan.
13. Mix all ingredients and put in greased casserole dish.
14. Sprinkle top with grated Parmesan and bake about 1 hour and 15 minutes at 350 degrees, until set and fork comes out clean.

Chicken & Zucchini Lasagna With White Sauce

Serves: 3

Ingredients

- 1 medium sized zucchini, sliced horizontally
- 3 ounces boneless and skinless chicken breast or thigh, chopped into big slices
- 1/8 cup olive oil
- 6 ounces chicken broth, low sodium
- 1 medium onion, finely chopped
- 1/4 teaspoon ground black pepper
- 1/2 tablespoon fresh or dried oregano
- 1/8 cup white wine (optional)
- 1 1/2 tablespoons flour
- 1/4 cup mushrooms, chopped into thick slices
- 3 ounces cream cheese
- 1/4 teaspoon nutmeg
- 3/4 cup non-dairy creamer, such as mocha mix
- 1/4 cup fresh parmesan cheese, grated
- 1 package no boil lasagna noodles

Preparation

1. Turn up your oven to 375 F (about 190 C) and preheat for about 10 to 20 minutes.
2. Pour the chicken broth and add the chicken breast slices into a small saucepan and heat over a high flame until lightly bubbling.

3. Reduce the heat and simmer and continue cooking until the chicken becomes white and is done.
4. While the chicken is simmering in the broth, you can heat some olive oil in a large sauté pan over a medium high flame. Then add the onion, ground black pepper and oregano to the pan and sauté for about 7 minutes or until the onion gets translucent and tender.
5. Add the wine (if using) to the pan and heat until the wine completely evaporates from the pan.
6. Add in the mushroom slices and toss the contents of the pan a few times for even cooking.
7. Sprinkle the flour over the contents of the pan and stir well. The contents of the pan should look clumpy.
8. Continue cooking for about 5 more minutes.
9. Crumble the cream cheese and add to the pan. Stir well and cook for about 3 minutes or until the cheese melts completely.
10. Slowly pour in the nondairy creamer and stir well to combine.
11. Keep heating until the sauce thickens. If the sauce is still lumpy, break apart the clumps and stir well to incorporate.
12. Sprinkle the nutmeg and mix well.
13. Add in the Parmesan cheese and stir continuously while cooking for about 5 minutes or until the sauce thickens.
14. Once the chicken is done strain it from the broth and shred it into even pieces using two forks. Set aside.

15. Pour about half of the chicken broth into the pan with the sauce and stir well until the sauce thins out. Cook for about 2 minutes, stirring occasionally.
16. Grease a square baking dish and place the no cook lasagna sheets in the bottom of the baking dish in a single layer. Ensure that the lasagna sheets do not overlap.
17. Pour about 1/3 of the prepared sauce over the lasagna sheets, and spread it in a thick even layer.
18. Add about half the shredded chicken over the sauce and distribute into a single even layer.
19. Spread about half the zucchini rounds in a single layer over the chicken.
20. Repeat the layers in the same order again: lasagna sheets, 1/3 sauce, shredded chicken, zucchini rounds and pour the remaining sauce over the zucchini rounds.
21. Cover the baking dish with a foil and pop into the preheated oven and bake for about 30 minutes.
22. Carefully remove the foil from the baking dish and broil for a few minutes without the foil until the sauce gets the desired level of crispiness.
23. Remove from the oven and serve immediately.
24. Enjoy!

Delicious Low Sodium Surf And Turf Gumbo

Serves: 6 (1 cup per serving)

Ingredients

- 1/2 tablespoon canola oil
- 1/2 yellow onion, finely chopped
- 2 celery stalks, finely chopped
- 1/2 red bell pepper, finely chopped
- 4 ounces lean turkey sausage, smoked and thinly sliced
- 1 skinless and boneless chicken breast, chopped into bite sized portions
- 1/4 cup canola oil
- 1/2 tablespoon Cajun seasoning (salt free)
- 1/4 cup flour
- 1 quart chicken broth, low sodium
- 3 ounces canned crab, drained
- 1/4 pound shrimp, cooked
- 1 1/2 cups frozen okra, finely chopped

Preparation

1. Pour the ½ tablespoon canola oil into a large pot, about 4 quart or more, and heat over a medium high flame.
2. Add the yellow onion, celery, red bell pepper, smoked turkey sausage, and chicken to the pot. Cook for about 10 minutes or until the celery, onion

and bell pepper are tender and the turkey sausage and chicken are cooked through.
3. Spoon out the mixture from the pot into a large mixing bowl and set aside.
4. Pour the ¼ cup canola oil into the pot and heat for a minute. Add in the flour and cook over a low flame, stirring constantly, to make a roux.
5. Add in the salt free Cajun seasoning and cook for a minute more, or even longer if you want the gumbo to have a dark color.
6. Slowly pour in the chicken broth, stirring constantly to ensure that no lumps form.
7. Once the roux and chicken broth are well incorporated, increase the heat and keep cooking until the mixture is bubbling. Lower the heat and simmer until the broth thickens slightly.
8. Add in the crab, okra, and shrimp and mix well.
9. Empty the chicken mix from the bowl back into the pot.
10. Turn the heat to the lowest setting, and cover the pot.
11. Let the broth simmer for at least 30 minutes.
12. Pour into individual bowls and serve immediately.
13. Enjoy!

Pan Cooked Chicken, Vegetable & Rice

Serves: 2

Ingredients

- 1/2 boneless, skinless chicken breast, cut into bite sized pieces
- 1 tablespoon + 1 tablespoon, divided olive oil
- 2 ears of corn, kernels removed from the cob
- 1/2 fresh zucchini, diced in cubes
- 1/2 red onion, finely diced
- 1/2 red bell pepper, diced in cubes
- 1/4 teaspoon garlic powder
- 1/4 teaspoon crushed black pepper
- 1/2 tablespoon cumin
- 2 cups rice, cooked
- 1 teaspoons Mrs. Dash original seasoning blend
- 1/4 teaspoon cayenne pepper

Preparation

1. Pour 1 tablespoon of olive oil into a large Teflon coated skillet and heat over a medium high flame.
2. Once the oil is hot, place the chicken pieces in the skillet. Stir well and cook for about 15 minutes or until the juices run clear.
3. Remove the chicken from the pan and set aside.
4. Pour the remaining oil into the skillet and heat it up.

5. Once hot, add in the corn, red pepper, zucchini and onion.
6. Sauté on a medium high flame for about 12 minutes or until the onions start to lightly caramelize. (Do not brown onions completely.)
7. Add in the garlic powder, crushed black pepper, cumin, cayenne pepper and Mrs. Dash original seasoning blend to the pan. Mix well.
8. Add the chicken back into the skillet and cook on a low flame for about 5 minutes, stirring constantly.
9. Add in the cooked rice and sauté for a couple of minutes until everything is well combined.
10. Serve immediately.
11. Enjoy!

Melt In The Mouth Crab Cakes

Serves: 4

Ingredients

- 2 cups crab meat, (drain the water)
- 1/4 cup celery, finely chopped
- 1/2 red bell pepper, finely chopped
- 1/4 cup onion, finely diced
- 1 egg
- 1/4 lemon juice
- 1/4 teaspoon hot pepper sauce
- 1/2 teaspoon Worcestershire sauce
- 1/2 tablespoon chives, minced
- 1/2 teaspoon fresh garlic, minced
- 1/2 teaspoon fresh thyme, minced
- 1/2 cup mayonnaise
- 3/4 cup panko crumbs

Preparation

1. Place the crabmeat, celery, chives, red bell pepper, garlic, thyme and onion together in a large mixing bowl.
2. Mix well using your fingers to properly combine.
3. In another bowl, whisk together the mayonnaise, egg, lemon juice, hot pepper sauce and Worcestershire sauce together until well blended.

4. Pour the prepared mayonnaise and sauce mix onto the crabmeat and vegetable mix and combine well using your fingers.
5. Pour the panko breadcrumbs into a flat plate or a flat baking sheet.
6. Spoon out a little scoop of the crabmeat mix and place on the panko breadcrumbs. Cover the crabmeat scoop in some panko breadcrumbs and slowly shape it into a cake.
7. Repeat with the remaining batter.
8. Place the crab cakes in a single layer in a plate and cover.
9. Refrigerate for at least 2 to 3 hours.
10. Pour some olive oil into a Teflon coated pan and heat over a medium high flame.
11. Place a few crab cakes into the hot oil and let the crab cake cook until heated thoroughly and golden brown on the outside. Repeat with the other side.
12. Once done, remove the crab cake from the pan and place on a kitchen towel to drain off the excess oil.
13. Serve hot with the sauce of your choice.
14. Enjoy!

Sweet & Spicy Honey Mustard Chicken

Serves: 2

Ingredients

- 2 tablespoons Dijon mustard
- 1/2 teaspoon curry powder
- 4 skinless and boneless chicken breasts
- 2 tablespoons honey
- 1/2 teaspoon lemon juice

Preparation

1. In a small mixing bowl, whisk together the honey and lemon juice until well combined.
2. Add in the Dijon mustard and the curry powder and whisk well.
3. Place the chicken in a large mixing bowl and pour the prepared marinade over the chicken.
4. Refrigerate for about 2 hours so that the chicken is well marinated.
5. Turn up your oven to 350 F (about 175 C) and preheat for about 10 to 20 minutes.
6. Place the marinated chicken in an oven safe pan and brush both sides of the chicken with the leftover marinade.
7. Pop into the preheated oven and bake for about 30 to 45 minutes or until the chicken is cooked through.

8. Remove the pan from the oven and let the chicken rest in the juices for about 5 minutes, before slicing it.
9. Serve hot.
10. Enjoy!

Pickled Carrots With Dill Weed

Serves: 2

Ingredients

- 1/2 pound carrots
- 1/4 cup plain rice vinegar
- 1 cup white vinegar
- 1 teaspoons dill weed
- 1/4 teaspoons pepper
- 2 tablespoons sugar
- 2 teaspoons garlic powder or fresh garlic, minced

Preparation

1. Wash the carrots vigorously and peel them. Cut them into thin sticks.
2. Heat a pot of water over a high flame. Once bubbling, lower the heat so that the water is simmering and place the carrots in a steaming basket or a sieve.
3. Cover and steam the carrots for about 5 to 7 minutes.
4. Once done, dunk the carrots into a bowl of ice water and drain.
5. Pat dry the carrots to get rid of excess water.
6. Combine the rice vinegar and white vinegar in a small mixing bowl. Whisk well to combine.
7. Add in the dill weed, pepper, sugar and garlic powder (or minced fresh garlic) and mix well.

8. Pour the prepared dressing over the steamed carrots and cover the bowl with a sling film.
9. Refrigerate overnight.
10. Serve chilled.
11. Enjoy!

Baked Fish With Lemon & Dill Weed

Serves: 1

Ingredients

- 2 teaspoons lemon juice
- 1 pound fresh white fish fillets
- 1/4 teaspoon mustard powder
- ½ teaspoon minced dry onion
- 1/2 teaspoon dill weed
- Crushed black pepper, to taste

Preparation

1. Turn up your oven to 475 F (about 250 C) and preheat for about 10 to 20 minutes.
2. Rinse the fish well and pat it dry with a kitchen towel.
3. Place the fish fillets, skin side down, in a greased baking dish.
4. Mix together the mustard powder, dry onion, dill, and pepper with about 1 tablespoon of water. Mix well.
5. Pour in the lemon juice and whisk well to combine.
6. Pour the prepared spice mix over the fish fillets.
7. Pop the baking dish into the preheated oven and bake uncovered for about 15 to 25 minutes.
8. Serve hot with a side of pan tossed vegetable.
9. Enjoy!

Zesty Grilled Chicken Kebabs With Lemon

Serves: 1

Ingredients

- 2 pieces skinless and boneless chicken thighs
- 2 tablespoons olive oil
- 2 lemons
- 1/2 clove garlic, peeled and crushed
- 1 bay leaf, torn in half
- 1/2 tablespoon chopped fresh herbs of your choice (such as, thyme, sage, basil, etc.)
- 1/2 teaspoon white wine vinegar

Preparation

1. Roughly chop up the chicken thighs into bite seized chunks and place in a large mixing bowl.
2. Zest one lemon and retrieve about ½ teaspoon worth of zest. Juice the lemon.
3. Pour the lemon juice over the chicken thighs and add the zest to it.
4. Pour the oil over the chicken breasts and add in the garlic, vinegar, bay leaf and herbs of your choice.
5. Mix well and cover with a cling film. Refrigerate for at least 3 hours to ensure proper marinating.
6. Chop the other lemon to get 4 thick slices. Then chop each slice into 4 additional pieces.

7. Skewer the lemon slices and chicken pieces alternatingly, starting and ending with a lemon. Pack as tightly as you can.
8. Grill on a BBQ, oven or a counter top grill for about 10 minutes on each side or until cooked.
9. Serve hot with your favorite dipping sauce.
10. Enjoy!

Chapter 8: Dessert Recipes

Crunchy Popcorn, Pecan And Almond Caramel

Serves: 5

Ingredients

- 6 tablespoons un-popped popcorn kernels
- 1/2 teaspoon baking soda
- 1/2 cup pecan halves
- 1 cup unblanched almonds, silvered
- 1/2 cup granulated sugar
- 1/4 cup corn syrup
- 1/2 cup unsalted butter
- A pinch of cream of tartar

Preparation

1. Combine together the un-popped popcorn kernels, silvered almonds and pecan halves in a medium sized mixing bowl.
2. Layer this mix into the bottom of a large roasting pan.
3. Turn up your oven to 200 F (about 100 C) and preheat for about 10 to 20 minutes.
4. In another heavy bottomed saucepan, place the corn syrup, sugar, butter and cream of tartar. Heat the pan on a high flame, stirring constantly, until the caramel is bubbling.

5. Allow the mixture to bubble for about 5 minutes, without stirring.
6. Take the pan off the heat and add in the baking soda. Mix well.
7. Pour the prepared caramel over the popcorn layer and toss to coat.
8. Pop the pan into the preheated oven and bake for about an hour.
9. Every 10 minutes, carefully open the oven, pull the pan out and give the ingredients a stir. This will ensure even roasting and will prevent the bottom or the top from burning.
10. Once done, remove from oven and cool. Stir it occasionally while it cools.
11. Serve immediately.
12. If you wish to store it, place it in an airtight container, away from direct sunlight. Do not store it for more than a week.
13. Enjoy!

Delicious & Nutty Baked Asian Pear Crisp

Serves: 4

Ingredients

- 6 tablespoons nuts of your choice, chopped
- 1/4 cup unbleached refined flour
- 2 tablespoons light brown sugar
- 1 tablespoon + 1 tablespoon white sugar
- 1/4 teaspoon ground cinnamon
- 1/8 teaspoon ground nutmeg
- 1/2 juice from lemon
- 1/2 tablespoon cornstarch
- 2 pounds Asian pears
- 3 tablespoons unsalted butter

Preparation

1. Turn up your oven to 375 F (about 190 C) and preheat for about 10 to 20 minutes.
2. Combine the chopped nuts, 1 tablespoon white sugar, brown sugar, nutmeg and cinnamon together in the jar of a blender.
3. Melt the butter in a microwave and pour it into the jar of the blender. Blitz until well combined and it looks like wet sand.
4. In a large bowl, whisk together the remaining 1 tablespoon white sugar, lemon juice and cornstarch, using a wire whisk.

5. Remove the peels of the pears, and remove the cores. Cut the pear into quarters, and halve those too.
6. Place the pears in the bowl with sugar and lemon mixture and toss well to coat.
7. Grease an 8-inch square baking dish with some oil. Layer the pears in the bottom of the baking dish.
8. Pour the nut mix from the blender jar over the pears.
9. Pop into the preheated oven and bake for about 50 minutes or until the fruit is bubbly around the edges and the nut mix gets a deep brown hue.
10. Remove from the oven and allow it to cool on a wire rack for about 15 minutes.
11. Serve immediately.
12. Enjoy!

Fresh Blueberry Cheesecake

Serves: 8

Ingredients

- 1 cup fresh blueberries, cut into quarters
- 1 cup Graham cracker crumbs
- ½ cup (4 ounces) Cream cheese, softened
- 1/4 cup Unsalted butter, melted
- 1/4 cup Granulated sugar
- 1 teaspoons lemon juice
- 1/2 teaspoon Vanilla extract
- ½ cup nondairy whipping cream

Preparation

1. Combine the graham cracker crumbs and the melted butter together in a small mixing bowl until it resembles wet sand.
2. Press this mix in the bottom of a greased 7-inch round baking pan. Press it down with your fingers so that it forms an even layer.
3. In a large mixing bowl place the cream cheese and sugar together. Using an electronic blender, whisk well until the cream cheese and sugar form a smooth paste.
4. Pour in the lemon juice and vanilla extract and mix well.
5. Gently pour in the whipped topping and cut and fold using a spatula.

6. Add in the blue berries and mix well with the spatula.
7. Spread this mixture evenly over the graham cracker crust and smoothen it using a spatula.
8. Cover with a cling film and chill for at least 4 to 6 hours, or even overnight if possible.
9. Cut it into 8 even slices and serve topped with some fresh blueberries.
10. Enjoy!

Quick & Easy Egg Caramel Custard

Serves: 3

Ingredients

- 1 tablespoon Sugar
- 3 Eggs
- 1 tablespoon Water
- 2 drops Vanilla extract
- 2 cups 2% milk
- 5 tablespoons Sugar

Preparation

1. To prepare the caramel place the sugar and water in a small saucepan and heat over a high flame until the sugar is caramelized and gets a pale golden color. This should take about 4 to 5 minutes.
2. You can also make caramel in a microwave. Place the sugar in a microwave safe container and pour the water over it.
3. Place the container in the microwave and set it at high power for about 4 minutes. Keep repeating until the sugar caramelizes.
4. Pour this caramel into the bottom of 3 soufflé ramekins.
5. Let the caramel cool to room temperature.
6. Turn up your oven to 350 F (about 175 C) and preheat for about 10 to 20 minutes.

7. To prepare the custard, crack the eggs in a medium sized mixing bowl.
8. Whisk by hand or use an electronic blender to whisk the eggs until they double in volume and get a frothy consistency.
9. Pour in the vanilla extract and continue whisking for a minute.
10. Slowly, add in the sugar, a little at a time and whisk until combined.
11. Similarly, pour in the milk and whisk until well incorporated.
12. Pour this prepared custard over the cooled caramel.
13. Pop the soufflé ramekins into the preheated oven and bake for 45 to 50 minutes.
14. Remove the soufflé ramekins from the oven and let them cool for about 30 minutes or until they are set.
15. Dip a knife into warm water and loosen the custard from the edges of the ramekin.
16. Place a serving plate on top of the soufflé ramekin and invert it over. If the caramel custard doesn't release from the soufflé ramekin, give it a gentle shake.
17. Serve immediately topped with some fresh fruit, such as, blueberries, banana slices, strawberries, orange rings, raspberries, etc.
18. Enjoy!

Chinese Style Vanilla Sponge Cake

Serves: 2

Ingredients

- 1/8 teaspoon baking powder
- 1 large egg
- 1/4 teaspoon vanilla
- 1/4 cup granulated sugar
- 1/4 cup all-purpose flour, sifted

Preparation

1. Turn up your oven to 325 F (about 150 C) and preheat for about 10 to 20 minutes.
2. Fill a pan halfway with water and place it inside the middle rack in the oven.
3. Line 2 ramekins with parchment paper.
4. Crack open the egg in a medium sized bowl and beat on low speed for about 10 minutes.
5. Once the egg is frothy, add in the sugar gradually, mixing well after each addition.
6. Once the sugar is incorporated, pour in the vanilla extract and continue beating.
7. Sieve in the flour and baking powder into the egg mixture and fold by hand until it forms a smooth batter.
8. Pour the prepared batter into the lined ramekins, until the halfway mark.

9. Place the ramekins into the water bath and bake for about 30 to 45 minutes or until a skewer poked in the center of the cake comes out clean.
10. Carefully remove the ramekins from the water bath and cool for about 10 minutes.
11. Remove the cake from the ramekin and cool on a wire rack.
12. Serve with topping of your choice.
13. Enjoy!

Mint Infused Chocolate Cake

Serves: 8

Ingredients

- 4 ounces chocolate, unsweetened
- 2 cups all-purpose flour
- 1 tablespoon baking powder
- 2 cups sugar
- 1/2 cup margarine or butter, unsalted
- 3 eggs
- 2 cups skim milk
- 1/2 teaspoon peppermint extract

Preparation

1. Turn up your oven to 350 F (about 175 C) and preheat for about 10 to 20 minutes.
2. Grease a 10-inch round baking pan with some butter or cooking spray. Sprinkle a little flour into the pan and twirl it so that the pan is well floured. Tap out the excess flour.
3. Sift the baking powder and sugar together into a small mixing bowl.
4. In a large mixing bowl, beat the butter or margarine with an electronic blender until creamy.
5. Add in the un-sifted flour, and baking powder and sugar mix and keep beating at a medium speed until smooth.
6. Add in the eggs and beat well.

7. Trickle in the vanilla extract and continue beating for another minute.
8. Heat the chocolate over a double boiler until almost melted.
9. Take off heat and add in the skim milk and peppermint extract and mix well using a spatula.
10. Add the chocolate mix into the prepared batter and mix using the cut and fold method.
11. Pour the cake batter into the prepared baking dish.
12. Pop the baking dish into the preheated oven and bake for about 30 minutes or until the cake begins to pull away from the edges of the pan and a skewer poked in the center of the cake comes out clean.
13. Remove from oven and cool in the pan for about 15 minutes.
14. Remove the cake from the pan and cool on a wire rack.
15. Cut into slices and serve with toppings of your choice.
16. Enjoy!

Quick & Easy Lemon Yogurt Parfait With Blueberries

Serves: 2

Ingredients

- 1 cup no fat yogurt
- 1 cups Blueberries, fresh or frozen (thawed out), cut into halves or quarters
- 1 lemon, zest removed and juiced
- 5 Gingersnap biscuits, crumbled

Preparation

1. In a medium mixing bowl, pour the no fat yogurt and whisk with a wire whisk until the yogurt it smooth and there are no lumps.
2. Pour in the lemon juice and whisk well to combine.
3. Sprinkle the lemon zest over the lemon and yogurt mix and mix lightly.
4. Divide the chopped blueberries between two tall wine glasses or parfait glasses.
5. Spoon in half of the lemon yogurt mix into each glass.
6. Chill in the refrigerator for at least 2 to 3 hours.
7. Just before serving, sprinkle the gingersnap biscuit crumble into each glass.
8. Serve immediately.
9. Enjoy!

Nutty Chocolate Fudge

Serves: 12 (2 pieces per serving)

Ingredients

- 2 cups semi-sweet chocolate chips
- 1/2 teaspoon baking soda
- ¼ cup unsweetened chocolate, chopped fine
- 1/8 teaspoon salt
- 1 tablespoon vanilla extract
- 2 cups sweetened condensed milk
- 1 cup walnuts

Preparation

1. Spray the bottom of an 8-inch x 8-inch pan with some cooking spray and line it with some parchment paper or aluminum foil (preferred). Spray again with some cooking spray.
2. Heat water in a pot on a high flame. Once bubbling, lower the heat until the water is simmering, and place a double boiler on top of the pot. Ensure that the bottom of the double boiler doesn't touch the surface of the water.
3. Add the semi-sweet chocolate chips, unsweetened chocolate shavings, salt and baking soda to the double boiler. Heat until well mixed.
4. Add in the condensed milk and vanilla extract and mix well using a spatula.

5. Once the chocolate is almost melted, take the double boiler off the heat and keep mixing for about 2 minutes or until the chocolate melts completely.
6. Add in the walnuts and mix well.
7. Pour the prepared chocolate and nut mix into the prepared baking dish.
8. Pop into the refrigerator and refrigerate overnight.
9. Remove the fudge from the pan by lifting the aluminum foil from the baking dish.
10. Cut into about 24 squares (cut 12 rows across and 12 rows down).
11. Serve immediately or store in an airtight jar in the refrigerator.
12. Enjoy!

No Bake Spiced Pumpkin Pie

Serves: 8 (1 slice per serving)

Ingredients

- 1 5 inch baked pie shell
- 1/2 cup canned pumpkin
- 1 cup vanilla ice cream, softened but not melted
- 1/2 cup sugar (can be adjusted to taste)
- 1/2 cup whipped topping
- 1/4 teaspoon cinnamon
- 1/4 teaspoon ginger
- 1/4 teaspoon nutmeg

Preparation

1. Place the canned pumpkin and softened ice cream in a large mixing bowl. Blend using a hand blender to form a smooth paste like consistency.
2. Add in the sugar, cinnamon, ginger and nutmeg and blend again.
3. Pour in the whipped topping and mix by hand, ensuring that all the ingredients are well incorporated.
4. Pour the prepared mix into the baked pie shell and level using a spatula.
5. Freeze overnight.
6. Serve chilled, topped with some whipped topping or a pinch of nutmeg.
7. Enjoy!

Conclusion

With that recipe, we have come to the end of this book. I want to thank you for choosing this book.

I hope this book helped you understand what renal failure diet is all about. You would have understood by now that it isn't just about following a diet for ensuring the health of your kidneys. But you should also make certain lifestyle changes and make the renal failure diet a part of your daily life if you want to maintain the health of your kidneys in the long run.

Since kidneys are vital for the proper functioning of the human body, you need to take good care of them. The first step for having healthy kidneys would be to incorporate all that you have read about in this book. You should also make sure that these practices become a habit for you and you will definitely start to notice a positive change in your overall health!

Thank you and all the best!

Made in the USA
Lexington, KY
02 November 2016